AF497301

TREE OF LIFE

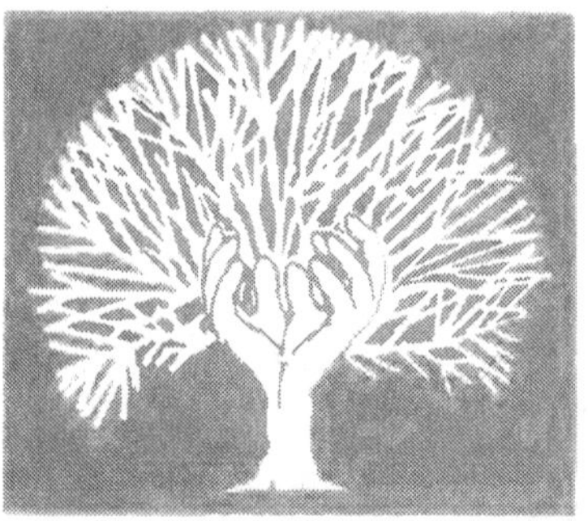

Transitional Housing For Homeless Women And Children

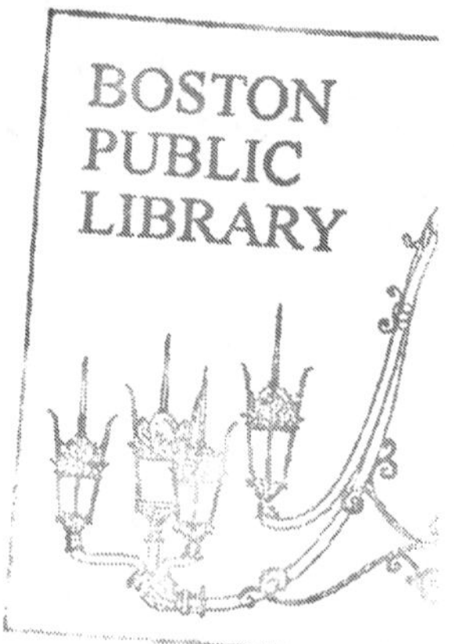

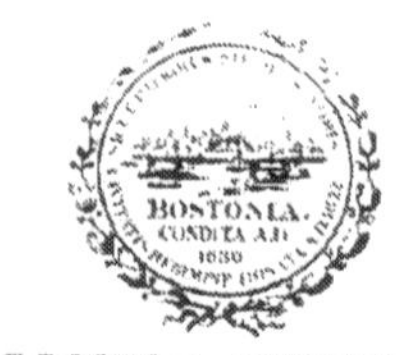

CITY OF BOSTON · MASSACHUSETTS

OFFICE OF THE MAYOR
RAYMOND L. FLYNN

Mr. Stephen Coyle
Director
Boston Redevelopment Authority
One City Hall Square
Boston, MA   02201

Dear Mr. Coyle:

As I have discussed with you, there is a growing need in our City for support housing for women and children. Over the past few years there has been an increase in the number of poor families headed by women. Domestic violence coupled with the shortage of affordable housing are the major contributors to this problem.

On countless evenings city government and social service agencies around the city receive requests from women and their children seeking shelter. On these evenings one is hard pressed to find any available shelter in the City. Further, if shelter is secured the length of stay is most often limited to a few weeks at most. Unless we are able to dramatically increase shelter for these families, many women will be forced to return to situations which threaten their safety and the safety of their children.

I would like the BRA to review potential sites and program models which can address this dire need. The program should focus on providing longer term housing, services and should assist as many families as possible. This program should be designed both comprehensively and compassionately.

Your prompt response to this request is appreciated.

Sincerely,

Raymond L. Flynn
Mayor of Boston

BOSTON
REDEVELOPMENT
AUTHORITY

Raymond L. Flynn
Mayor

Stephen Coyle
Director

One City Hall Square
Boston, MA 02201
(617) 722-4300

August 1, 1986

Honorable Raymond L. Flynn
Mayor of Boston
One City Hall Square
Boston, MA 02201

Dear Mayor Flynn:

This proposal is a response to your request for an innovative approach to
serving the needs of homeless women and children in Boston. The proposal
is transitional housing to provide shelter, employment training, health
services, and moral support necessary to help many women cross from a life
of dependency to a life of independence and self-sufficiency.

The key features of this proposal are:

o 100 units for homeless women and their children;
o 10,000 square feet of retail space to produce income for the operating
   costs of the program, and to provide potential employment opportunities
   for some of the women;
o The project would be financed by a variety of public and private sources,
   including city-owned land, voluntary linkage contributions, rental assistance programs, grants, and other private contributions;
o The design of the project is compatible with the surrounding neighborhood, and would contribute to the urban fabric of the area;
o Groundbreaking could occur in spring of 1987, with occupancy by 1988.

A project team of BRA staff has been assembled to handle the design, financial, legal, zoning, and planning analyses for the project. I have asked
Carole Pelletier of my staff to manage this team, and to work with members of
your Office to coordinate our efforts with other aspects of the overall program
development.

To date, we have met with key representatives of the provider community to
elicit their support and input into the program. I was heartened by their
positive reception to your idea, and by their willingness to help us gain
broader community support.

With your leadership and direction, we will continue to work toward the
fulfillment of a project that will stand as a symbol of your concern for the
plight of homeless people; and will serve the needs of a desperate segment of
Boston residents.

Sincerely,

Stephen Coyle
Director

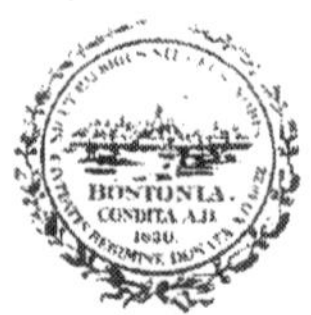

CITY OF BOSTON · MASSACHUSETTS

OFFICE OF THE MAYOR
RAYMOND L. FLYNN

August 5, 1986

Carolyn Gritter
Chairwoman
Women's Commission
City of Boston
One City Hall Square
Boston, MA 02201

Dear Ms. Gritter:

I would like to inform the Women's Commission of a very important program which the City will be embarking upon; a program where the input and expertise of the Women's Commission will be needed.

As you well know, the number of women with children who are in need of support housing is growing. Family shelters throughout the City are full each night. Physical and sexual abuse are prime factors in this growing problem. I have directed the Boston Redevelopment Authority and other City officials to site and develop a comprehensive and compassionate transitional housing program for these women and their children.

Much work needs to be done in order for this program to be successful. The assistance of the Women's Commission will be essential if we are to develop a plan which understands and fully addresses the problems which face these families. We will be working with the community to educate them on this proposal. We also will be seeking guidance from providers and the social service agencies on how best to develop this program. The assistance of the Women's Commission in each of these endeavors will be instrumental.

Again, I want to stress the importance of this program to our City and thank you in advance for your efforts.

Sincerely,

Raymond L. Flynn
Mayor of Boston

MEMO
TO·   MAYOR FLYNN
FROM: SUSAN TRACY *SMT*
DATE: AUGUST 7, 1986
RE·   OUTREACH DONE ON PROPOSED TRANSITIONAL HOUSING FOR WOMEN & CHILDREN

We have begun discussions with members of the shelter provider community to seek their input and ideas on the City's proposed transitional housing for women and children.

As you know, on August 6th, you and members of your staff met with Rich Ring and Father McLaughlin of the Emergency Shelter Commission. Fr McLaughlin operates Crossroads, a family shelter in East Boston, which runs at capacity each evening. Fr. McLaughlin recognizes the great need for increasing our services for this population and gave his support and commitment to the proposal. Rich Ring of the Pine Street Inn stressed that, apart from meeting the needs of the deinstitutionalized mentally ill homeless, increasing the supply of transitional housing is one of our greatest needs. Ring, too, offered his assistance in helping to make these efforts a success.

Last week Nancy Snyder, BRA staff and I met with Joan Sprague of the Women's Institute for Housing and Economic Development and with Val Lanier and Ann Slattery of the Paul Sullivan Housing Trust. Joan Sprague has published a manual on transitional housing and Val Lanier and Ann Slattery have been responsible for siting and developing such housing for the Sullivan Trust.

Sprague, Lanier and Slattery were enthused about the project. They all recognize the immense need for such a program and offered their support for the proposal. They stressed the importance of having strong management at the site and of trying to educate the community about the benefits and importance of the program.

Presently we are compiling a list of leaders in the homeless community, in particular those who work with women and children, to meet with us next week to be briefed on the plans.

The Office of Neighborhood Services will also begin discussions with the community next week.

<u>Executive Summary</u>

o   The Tree of Life would provide transitional housing for 100 homeless
    women and their children   Transitional housing provides shelter for
    up to two years   During that time, women would receive counseling, job
    training, health services and community support as needed to help them
    cross from a life of dependency to a life of independence and self-
    sufficiency   Transitional housing programs have been successfully
    established across the nation

o   The design concept of the Tree of Life residences is compatible with the
    architecture of the South End neighborhood   Ground floor retail activity
    along Washington Street would be convenient to area residents   Franklin
    and Blackstone Squares, two of the oldest parks in the South End, are
    located close to the Tree of Life site

o   Financing for the development and operation of the Tree of Life project
    would come from a variety of public, private, and philanthropic sources
    Total development cost is estimated at around $12 million   It is expected
    that operating income from the project would be able to support the
    project's debt service payments   State and federal rental subsidies and
    social service programs would be sought to support program operating
    costs   Voluntary developer contributions, private contributions from
    corporations, individuals, and philanthropic organizations, acquisition
    proceeds from other parcels, and sales proceeds from additional units
    built into the project would be available to defray upfront development
    costs

o   Groundbreaking for Tree of Life would be planned for the Spring of
    1987, to be completed and ready for occupancy in 1988

o   The Tree of Life would be owned and operated by a private, non-profit
    corporation   The Board of Directors of this corporation would be a
    combination of community residents, social service providers,
    representatives from the business community and others   All board
    members would be appointed by the Mayor

Table of Contents

1
Introduction

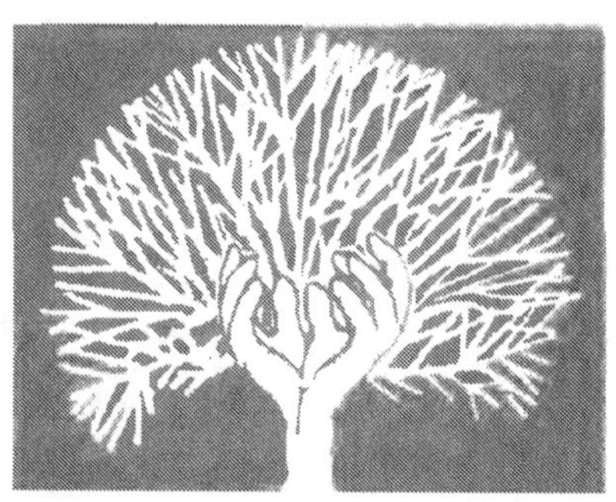

<u>Tree of Life</u>

<u>Transitional Housing For Homeless Women and Children</u>

The homeless population nationwide is growing In fact, more Americans were homeless this winter than at any time since the Great Depression In Boston, the number of homeless people is estimated to be between 3,000 and 5,000 Causes of homelessness, such as de-institutionalization and the growing number of single parent families, are compounded by the short supply of affordable rental housing units In Boston, where nearly 70% of all households rent, rents increased 18% to 31% annually between 1982 and 1985 The rental vacancy rate in Boston is currently below 3%, and the average waiting period for public housing is 5 years This tight housing market has added to the problem of homelessness in Boston, and has consequently led to the increased demands on the city's shelters

There are currently 100 Boston families living in emergency shelters, and an additional 100 homeless families living in hotels in and around the city Taking into account families that are are doubled up, and those remaining in a bad situation because they have nowhere else to go, the number of distressed families is much higher Family shelters in Boston report no vacancies Many shelters receive an average of 50 phone calls a month from families they are unable to accommodate For those families fortunate enough to be placed in a shelter, the vast majority are unable to locate a permanent residence by the end of 3 months

The characteristics and needs of Boston's homeless individuals and families are varied The facilities and services required to meet the needs of homeless people are also diverse Emergency shelters serve the vital function of providing immediate assistance to homeless people Most shelters,

however, are not designed to provide follow-up services for long term
stabilization Homeless people need continuing support and training to become
self-sufficient providers for themselves and for their children Emergency
shelters and longer term facilities complement each other, both are needed to
deal with the crisis of homelessness in this city.

Tree of Life is proposed as a transitional housing program targeted for a
special segment of the homeless population women and their children As
the number of homeless people has grown so has the percentage of women who
are homeless While the majority of homeless people are still men, the
increase in the number of women has been significant enough for some to call
it "the feminization of homelessness " This increase in the number of homeless women has paralleled the growth of female-headed households

During the last decade, the number of female-headed households nationwide
rose dramatically Whether through divorce, separation, widowhood, or
teenage motherhood, an increasing number of women found themselves as the
sole provider for their families In 1980, 30% of Boston's families were headed
by single women, 63% of those families had children under the age of 18 At
a time when women are emerging as major family providers, the number of
women and children living in poverty is also growing In Boston, 37% of
families headed by women live at or below the poverty line, for women with
children under 18, the percentage is an astonishing 53% Various economic
factors contribute to the plight of these families, including the severe shortage of affordable housing in the city, lack of job experience, shortage of
adequate childcare, and reduced welfare benefits

Boston's downtown economy is producing unprecedented opportunities for
the residents of the city, yet many low income women face barriers to
obtaining these opportunities Lack of adequate shelter, the need for

childcare, and the need to upgrade skills are among the types of assistance these women need to take advantage of job opportunities <u>Transitional housing</u> -- or multi-family residency programs -- provides the support and services that many homeless women need to attain self-sufficiency The development of a transitional housing facility would provide Boston's low income women and children with low cost shelter, childcare, counseling, legal assistance, job training, and career planning Women would receive this social service assistance in addition to the emotional and psychological support they need to begin rebuilding their lives Typically, women reside in transitional facilities for up to two years.

Importantly, this initiative would combine the resources and experience of the private sector, the public sector, and the community to provide a new transitional housing facility for Boston's homeless women and their children The housing facility proposed would accommodate 100 women and their families, with a childcare facility and outdoor space Women in the facility would receive job training, counseling, and medical care Financing for the development and operation of this project would come from a variety of sources, both public and private The resources of local businesses, government, and non-profit community-based groups would be used to extend the benefits of economic growth to those families most in need

The site selected for this transitional housing facility is Parcel RC-9, a 49,232 square foot parcel bounded by Shawmut Avenue, West Concord Street, Washington Street, and Rutland Street in the South End A portion of Parcels 30 and RD-60, totalling roughly 19,500 square feet, would also be used This combined site is located on the Washington Street Corridor, a main thoroughfare, and is currently near two subway stops After planned redevelopment is completed, a bus or trolley will run by the site

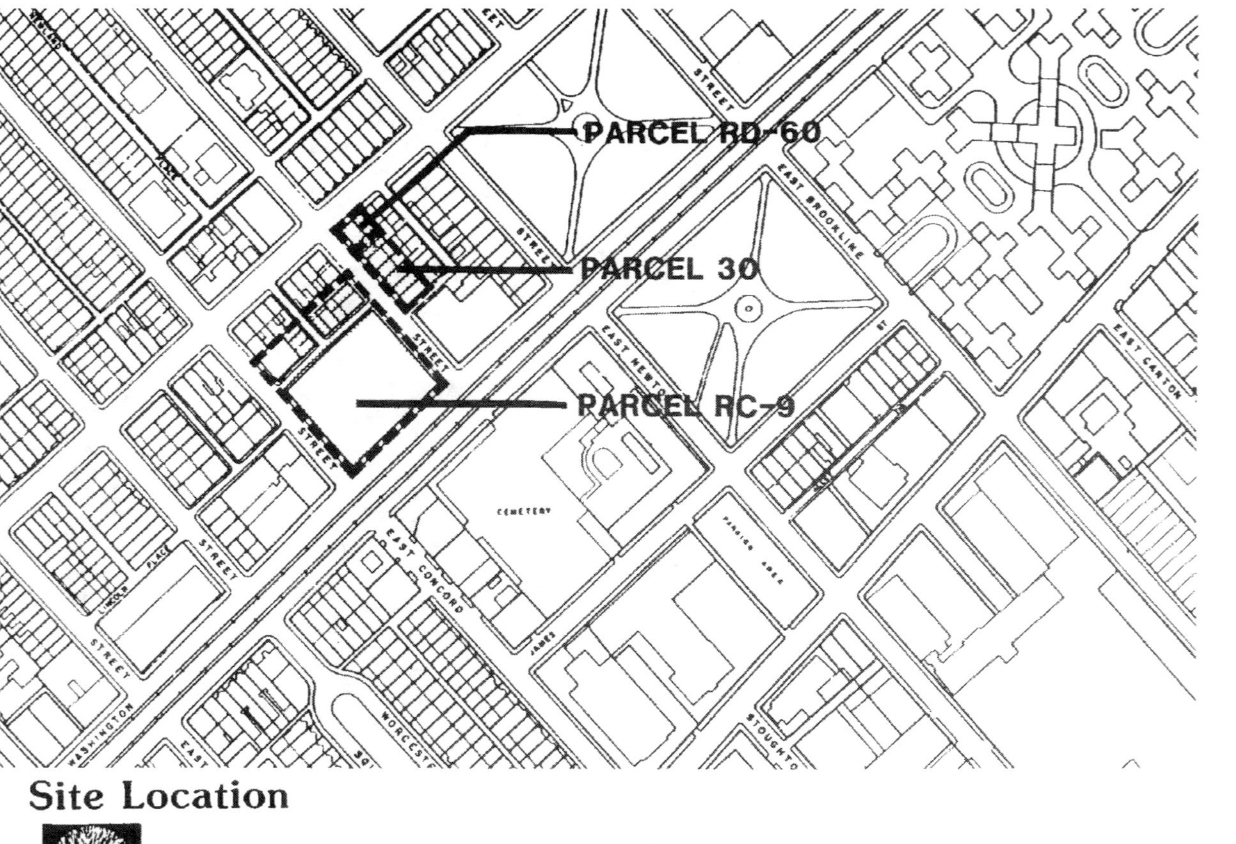

Site Location

TREE OF LIFE

Transitional Housing
Homeless Women And Children

Blackstone Square and Franklin Square, in close proximity to the site, are the oldest parks in the South End They have recently been rehabilitated according to their 1851 plans A victorian fence encircles each park and its fountains and benches Adjacent to parcel RC-9 is a garden and a newly constructed gazebo sponsored by the Boston Urban Gardeners Across from the site is the South End Burial Ground These greenspaces will provide ample recreational and open space for the children and their mothers

The Blackstone School, an elementary school, is nearby with its playground, library, and other resources The Boston City Hospital and Boston University Hospital are both easily accessible to the site The city will invest $173 million to reconstruct the in-patient facilities at Boston City Hospital, construction is scheduled to begin in 1987

2
Development Concept

<u>Development Concept</u>

Developed at a cost of roughly $12 million, the Tree of Life transitional housing project would be constructed on three BRA-owned parcels in the South End at Washington and Rutland Streets.

The current development proposal calls for the construction of a housing facility with a total of 76 units on Parcel RC-9, including 41 two- and three-bedroom family apartments of 1,200 GSF each, and 35 congregate living units of 800 GSF each   This development would also include a 4,000 GSF day care center for children of house residents, that could be operated and maintained as a separate entity   Additional space would be allocated for resident staff, administration services, and common areas   Most of the project's social services would be located off-site

In order to integrate the Tree of Life project into the surrounding neighborhood, 10,000 GSF of ground level retail would be included in the project   With rental rates at $15/GSF, the proposed retail space would generate $150,000 of income a year   The project would also have 32 parking spaces, approximately 20 of which could be rented to residents of the community Parking spaces could provide an additional $36,000 in annual income

This development scenario includes an additional 25 units of transitional housing on portions of Parcels 30 and RD-60, fronting on Rutland Avenue An additional 8 units (in 2 rowhouses) built to front on Shawmut Avenue would be sold for approximately $185,000 each, to help to defray initial start-up costs for the project

Under this proposal a total development cost of $12 million is expected An added 5% of hard costs has also been assumed to cover the establishment of a reserve or sinking fund to be used as needed during the project's

on-going operations   This reserve fund allocation, when added to the total
development cost, results in total project costs of $12 7 million   Construction
costs are estimated at $65/GSF for the transitional units, $70/GSF for the
condominiums, and $15/GSF for the site costs

Soft costs are expected to be obtained at cost from local architectural,
legal, and accounting firms providing pro bono services

Since each transitional living unit must be fully furnished, 10% of hard
costs has been allocated for furniture, fixtures, and equipment (FF&E)
These funds would be distributed proportionately to provide furnishings for
both the transitional housing units and corridor areas, kitchen facilities, day
care facilities, administrative and program spaces

Project Financing

Based on the assumed net operating income, the Tree of Life facility
could support a $5 million mortgage   While retail space, parking spaces, and
condominium unit sales would produce income to help fund the operating
expenses of the Tree of Life, outside financial assistance would be necessary
to cover the project's debt service and operational obligations   Federal grant
programs and state rental subsidies for the project have been identified and
will be pursued, in addition to private sector sources

A portion of BRA voluntary linkage contributions are presently earmarked
for the Tree of Life project, with some funds available as early as 1987   It
is proposed that the Tree of Life borrow against these monies   This remaining
gap could be financed in a number of ways including the possible sale of
other nearby parcels in the South End   Additional money could also be
raised through a citywide fundraising effort, targeting area business people,
philanthropists, and developers

DEVELOPMENT PROGRAM

Site Location:	RC-9		RD-60 and Parcel 30
Parcel Size (GSF):	49,232		19,491
Proposed GSF:		129,500	
Lot Coverage Ratio:	40.00%		

TRANSITIONAL HOUSING

Unit Type	# of Units	GSF Per Unit	GSF	Percent Efficiency	NSF
2&3 Bedroom/Family	66	1,200	79,200	90.00%	71,280
Congregate Living:	35	800	28,000	90.00%	25,200
Retail:			10,000	90.00%	9,000
Residential Staff Space:			1,600	90.00%	1,440
Administrative Space:			1,200	90.00%	1,080
Day Care Facilities (100SF/Child):			4,000	90.00%	3,600
Lobby & Halls:			3,500	98.00%	3,430
Kitchen Facilit.:			2,000	90.00%	1,800
TOTAL:	101		129,500		116,830

CONDOMINIUM DEVELOPMENT (Rutland & Shawmut Streets)

Unit Type	# of Units	GSF Per Unit	GSF	Percent Efficiency	NSF
2&3 Bedroom/Family	8	1,000	8,000	90.00%	7,200

SITE DEVELOPMENT:

On-Grade Parking:			
No. of Sapces:	32	Spaces for Hsg.	12
GSF/Space:	350	Spaces for Rent	20
TOTAL SQUARE FOOTAGE:11,200		Total Spaces	32

LANDSCAPED AREA: 18,339
  (Inc. tot lot)

TOTAL DEVELOPMENT SITE: 29,539

<u>Tree of Life</u>

<u>Transitional Housing for Homeless Women and Children</u>

<u>DEVELOPMENT PRO FORMA</u>

ACQUISITION COST:
Parcel: RC-9 $ 0

HARD COSTS:

	Cost/GSF	Cost
Construction:		
Housing:	$65	$ 7,767,500
Retail:	65	650,000
Condominium:	70	560,000
Site Costs (LSF):	15	443,088
TOTAL HARD COSTS:		**$ 9,420,588**

SOFT COSTS:

	Cost/GSF	Cost
Architecture/Engineering		$ 282,618
Percent of Hard Costs:	3.00%	
Legal & Prof. Fees:	1.00%	94,206
Construction Loan Interest (@11% for 1 year)		518,132
TOTAL SOFT COSTS:		**$ 894,956**

		Cost
Room, Kitchen, & Day Care Furniture, Fixtures, & Equipment (FE&E):	10.00%	$ 821,059
CONTINGENCY @10% of Hard Cost:		$ 942,059
TOTAL DEVELOPMENT COST:		**$12,078,661**

<u>NOTES</u>:

1. Many of the services associated with Soft Costs will be donated or provided at cost.

2. Acquisition cost of $0 is assumed to represent a nominal land acquisition cost.

3. It is assumed that the mortgage amount will be limited to $5,000,000.

4. All development and operating information included in these pro formas is based upon preliminary estimates.

<u>Tree of Life</u>

<u>Transitional Housing for Homeless Women and Children</u>

<u>DEVELOPMENT FUNDING</u>

Total Development Cost	$12,078,661
Reserve/Sinking Fund (5% of TDC)	603,933
Total Project Cost·	12,682,594
Condo TDC	680,000
Total less Condo	$12,002,594
Mortgage Limit	$ 5,000,000

TDC Gap	$ 7,002,594
Voluntary Contributions	2,250,000
TDC Gap	4,752,594
Income from Condos	740,800
Public Grant	2,000,000
TDC GAP	$ 2,011,794

<u>CONDOMINIUM SALES PRO FORMA</u>

Unit Price	$	185,000
Price/Square Foot		185
Gross Sales		1,480,000
Marketing/Brokerage Fee		59,200
Condo Dev Cost ($85/GSF)		680,000
Net Profit (pre-tax)	$	740,800
RETURN ON GROSS SALES PROCEEDS		50 05%

<u>Tree of Life</u>

<u>Transitional Housing for Homeless Women and Children</u>

<u>OPERATING FUNDING</u> - First Stabilized Year

	Income/Unit	Income
INCOME		
2 bedroom units (33)*	$ 718	$ 284,328
3 bedroom units (33)*	895	354,420
Congregate Space (35)	611	256,620
Retail (10,000 SF)	15 00	150,000
Parking		
(20 Spaces @ $150/month)		36,000
Day Care Income		
TOTAL GROSS INCOME		$1,081,368
Vacancy @ 3%		$ 32,441
EFFECTIVE GROSS INCOME		$1,048,927
EXPENSES		
Operating Expenses		
Housing Management		$ 48,480
Maintenance		48,480
Day Care Operation		
Staff - Social Services (13)		260,000
Overhead		35,000
Real Estate Taxes		
Utilities		75,144
Common Space/Staff Units		25,816
Replacement & Oper Reserve		25,250
Legal and Accounting		10,489
Insurance		67,641
Security		60,000
TOTAL EXPENSES		($656,299)
Social Services Contract		295,000
NET OPERATING INCOME		$ 687,628

3

Design Concept

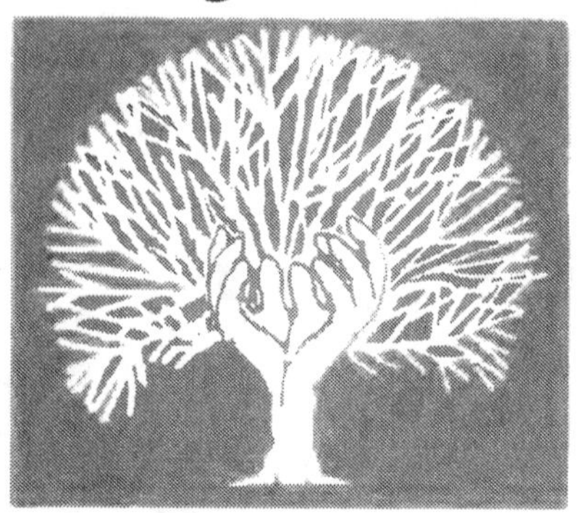

<u>Design Concept</u>

The Tree of Life project would provide 76 family dwelling units on
Parcel RC-9 in the South End An additional 25 families would be
accommodated across Rutland Street from Parcel RC-9 on a portion of
Parcel 30 north of Haven Street.

The development on RC-9 is conceived as a four and five story, brick,
U-shaped building with distinctly public and private aspects The public
facades wrap around the perimeter of the site along West Concord Street,
Washington Street and Rutland Street filling in large gaps in the South End
building fabric These facades are punctuated with bows and entry stoops to
relate to the historic Victorian rowhouses that predominate in the neighborhood A varied roofline helps to break down the massing of the building to a
residential scale Retail uses are provided at the ground floor along
Washington Street in order to strengthen its neighborhood commercial character

The private face on the inside of the U focuses on a shared open area to
provide a space for residents to relax and enjoy A tot lot is adjacent to the
day care center located on the ground floor along West Concord Street

The building itself can provide a range of alternative living arrange-
ments The concept illustrated here contains a mix of 2 and 3 bedroom
apartments for single families, and 4 to 5 family congregate units Some of
the apartments could have individual access from the street, others could be
accessed through a central lobby Every floor contains shared spaces for
informal meetings and interaction A central lobby/greenhouse overlooking

the green space provides a shared meeting place large enough to accommodate all residents   A large kitchen facility and food storage area is provided to accommodate a food co-operative and a large serving area for special events

The development on Parcel 30 is compatible with traditional South End rowhouses   Each one of these could house either a large congregate unit or more conventional two bedroom apartments on each floor   Parcel RD-60, which is contiguous to Parcel 30 directly to the north would be developed with two market rate rowhouses fronting on Shawmut Avenue

The Tree of Life project is designed to become an integral part of the South End community   It combines a needed social service with retail, open space, and buildings that are designed to accord with the South End Landmark District regulations   The design quality is geared towards fitting the project into its historic context; it also symbolizes the city's deep commitment toward this important social program

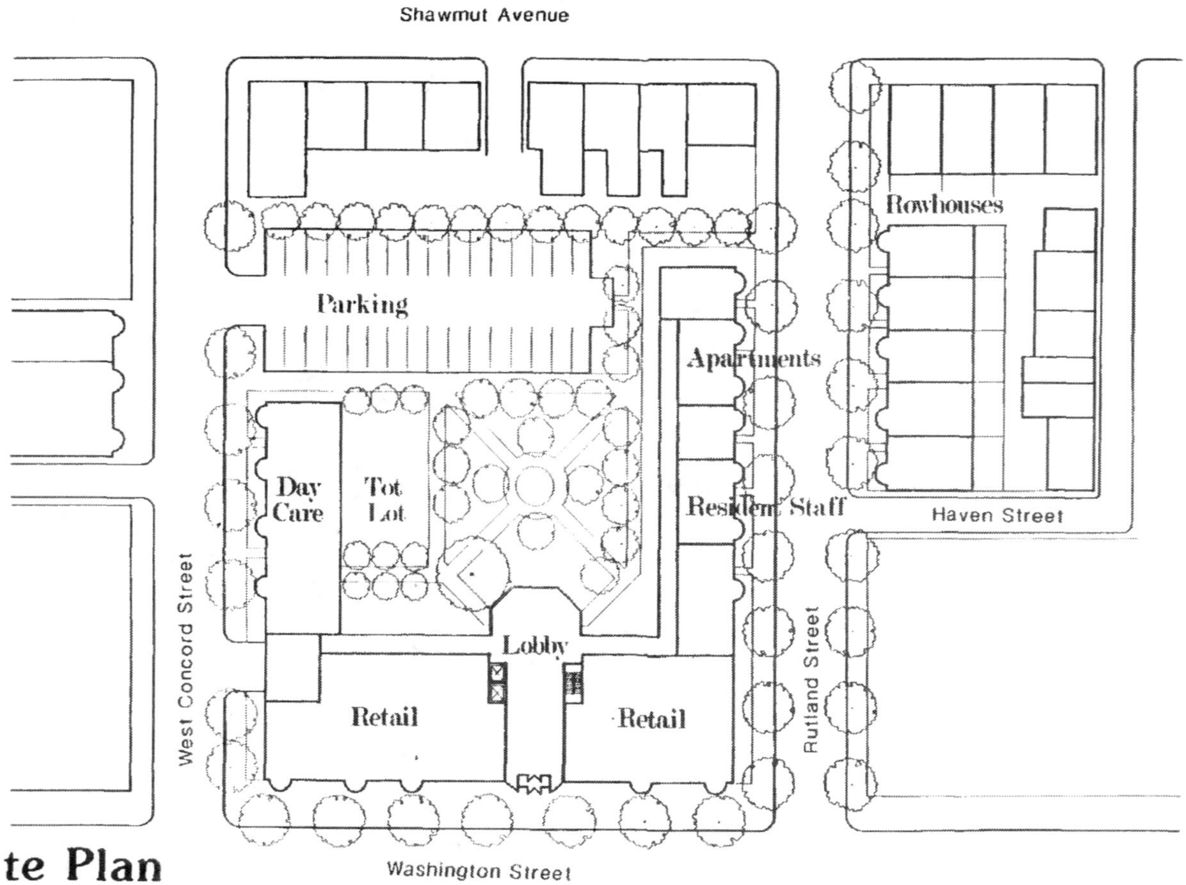

Site Plan

TREE OF LIFE

Transitional Housing
Homeless Women And Children

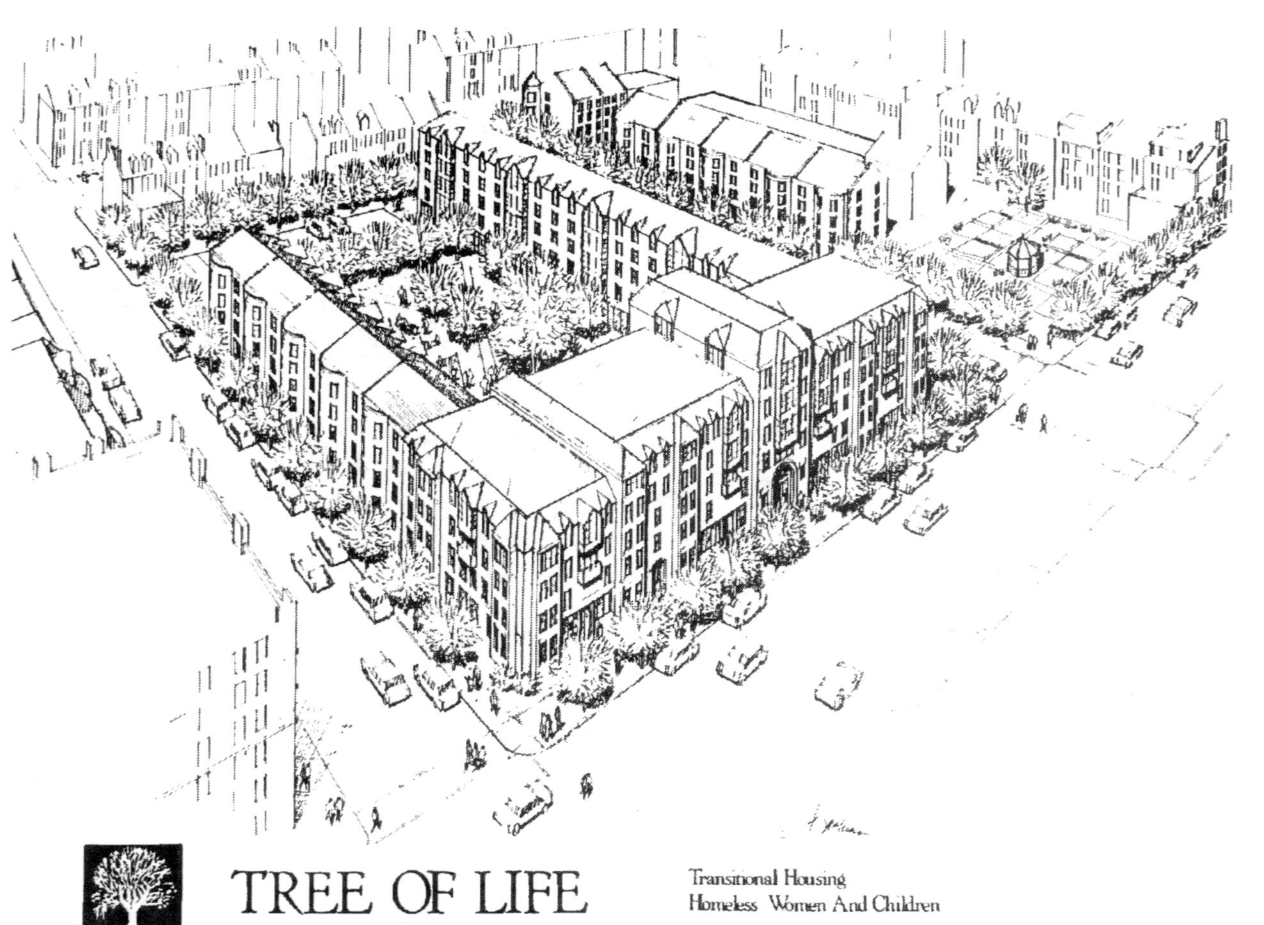

TREE OF LIFE
Transitional Housing
Homeless Women And Children

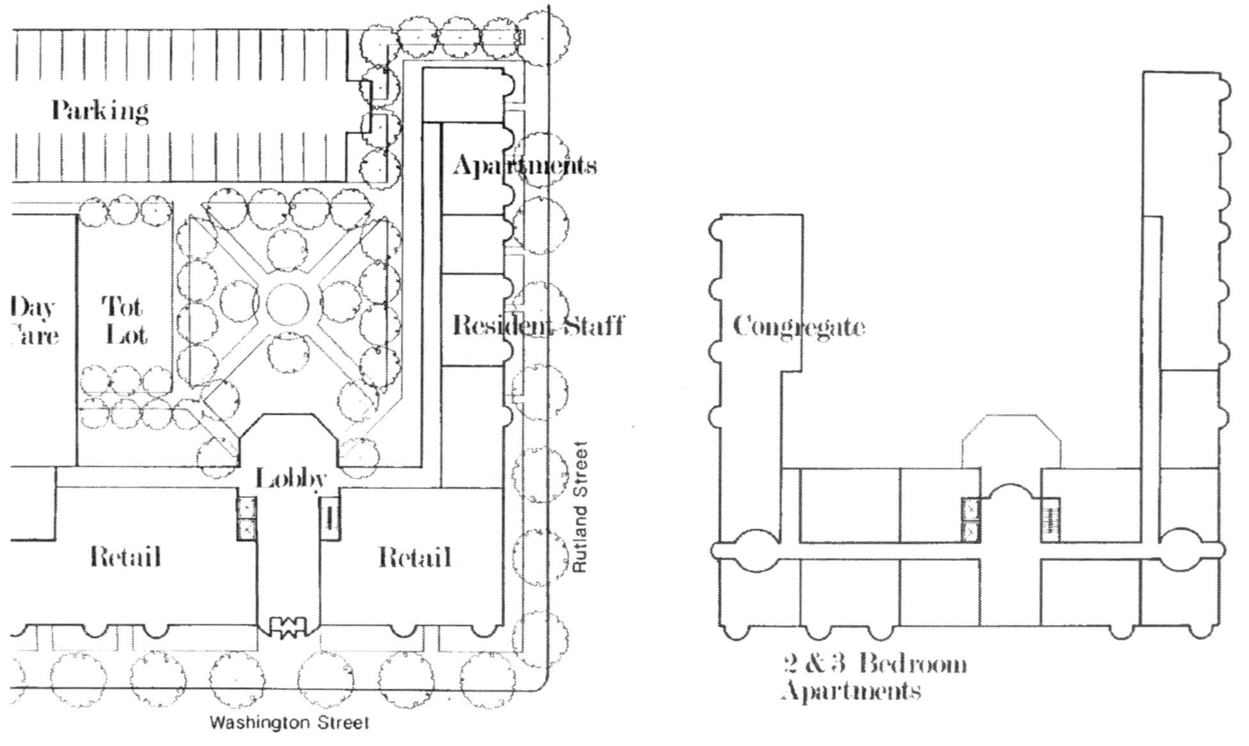

Ground Floor Plan

Upper Level Plan

TREE OF LIFE

Transitional Housing
Homeless Women And Children

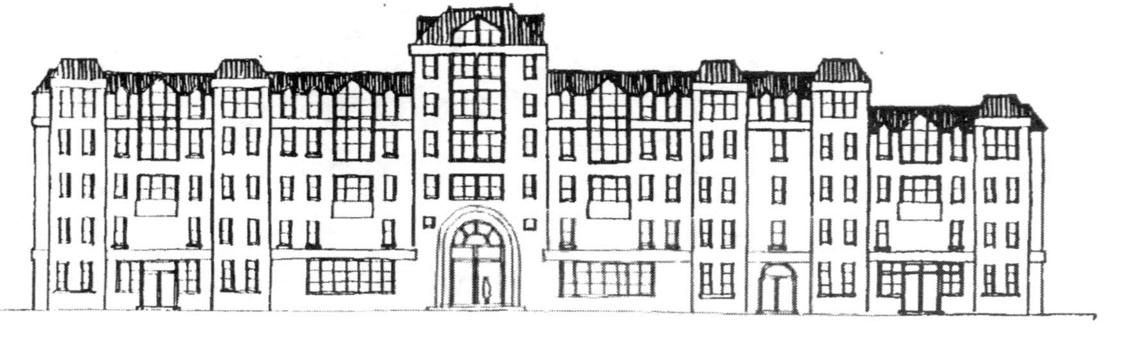

Front Elevation

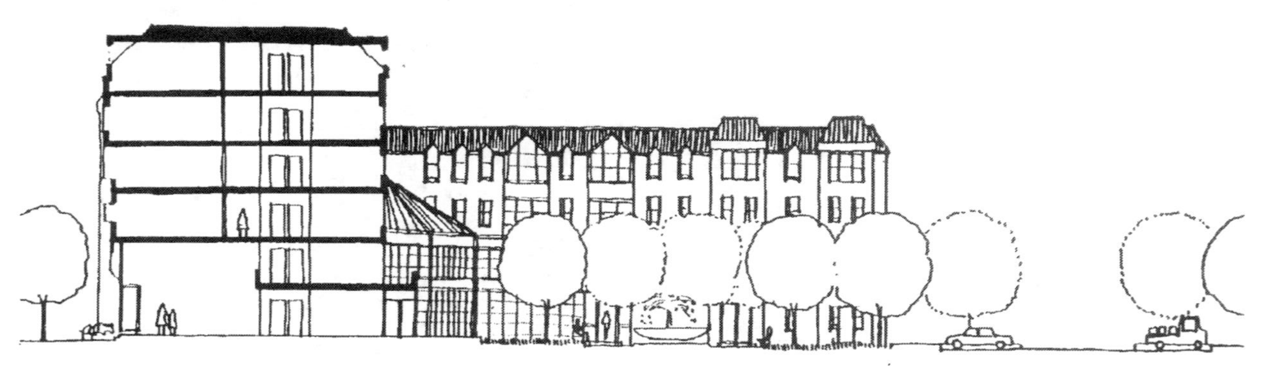

Section Through Lobby

TREE OF LIFE

Transitional Housing
Homeless Women And Children

4

Program Concept

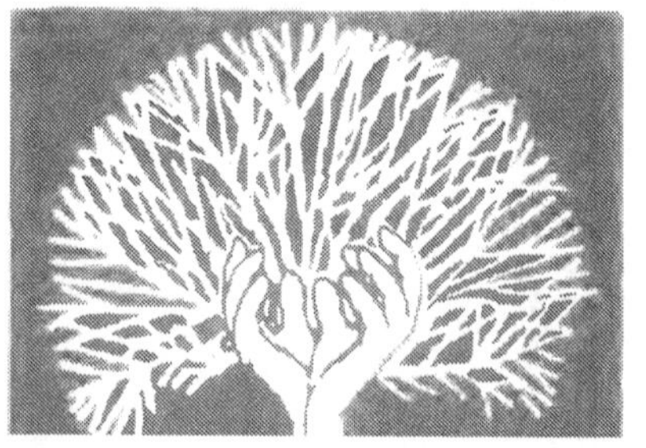

<u>Program Concept</u>

The concept of developing transitional housing depends upon the coordination of a broad range of social services to meet the needs of homeless women and their children The Tree of Life project would not only provide shelter but a supportive environment to women and their families as they adjust to an independent lifestyle Effective orientation for families entering the community requires a variety of activities and services in the areas of health, education, job-training, and housing These services will be provided either on-site or by nearby providers Neighborhood social service and health care agencies in the South End would play a key role in providing many of these vital services

o   The present development concept includes space for on-site daycare services for pre-school age children With a 4,000 GSF daycare center and a tot-lot, the center would be able to accommodate approximately 60 children

o   Living quarters have been set aside for live-in residential staff At least one staff person would be responsible for the management and maintenance of the buildings and rounds, other live-in staff would work more closely with the women overseeing day-to-day programmatic activities

o   Office space and meeting rooms would be provided for both full-time administrative staff, and for the provision of on-site services such as career counseling and job training

o   Networks with local hospitals and health care agencies would be established to facilitate psychological counseling, health care services, drug counseling, and other social services for residents

o   Security would be monitored through modern, state-of-the-art security systems Additional 24-hour building security may also be available

o   Women would be encouraged and assisted in the use of public transportation Additional transportation would be provided as necessary

<u>Development Entity and Affiliates</u>

The BRA-owned land on which the project would be built would be transferred by the Authority to an entity organized as a non-profit corporation under Chapter 180 of the Massachusetts General Laws, and under Section 501(C)(3) of the Internal Revenue Code This "Parent Corporation" would be formed by individuals selected by the Mayor, and he would have the authority to appoint the members on an annual basis In addition, the Parent Corporation would apply for designation by the Authority as a "121A" entity under Chapter 121A of the General Laws and the Acts of 1960, Chapter 652

There are several advantages to this structure. First, as a tax exempt non-profit entity, the Parent Corporation would be exempt from both federal and state income taxes Additionally, third parties would be entitled to federal and state charitable deductions for contributions and donations of in-kind services The Parent Corporation would have the responsibility to finance and construct the project All legal, architectural and development consultant services could be provided by professionals on a "pro bono" basis, or charitable deductions could be taken for the services rendered to the project Furthermore, the Parent Corporation could raise capital funds for construction of the project from individual donors or foundations

Second, as a "121A" entity, the Parent Corporation and the project would be exempt from local real estate taxes which would serve to minimize the project's tax burden Importantly, the BRA could grant necessary deviations from the Boston Zoning Code as part of its 121 approval This would eliminate the need to secure variances from the Zoning Board of Appeal

Upon completion of the project, the Parent Corporation would divide the facility into two segments, and lease the respective segments to affiliated entities as follows:

A   The housing/social services segment would be leased for nominal rent to another non-profit tax exempt corporation, which would be responsible for management ("Affiliate A") The Mayor would also have the authority to appoint the members of this corporation

B   The retail segment would be leased to a for-profit corporation ("Affiliate B") which would be a wholly-owned subsidiary of Affiliate A, the non-profit tax exempt corporation that operates the housing/social services segment The net income of Affiliate B would be paid to Affiliate A as an operating subsidy for its housing/social service activities.

Based on this proposed leasing structure, the Chapter 121A payments of the Parent Corporation, including both the annual payment to the state and the payments required by the City of Boston, would be minimized Since the gross income of the Parent Corporation is limited to is nominal rent under the proposed leases with Affiliates A and B, the payments would be limited to little more than one percent (1%) of the fair cash value of the project, as determined annually by the Assessing Department

A number of transitional housing programs are being developed and operated across the country These programs vary in many ways, including their size, the residents they serve, and the types of services they provide While none of these facilities is strictly a model for the Tree of Life, their experiences provide insight into the strengths and weaknesses of various program options

Warren Village

Warren Village is a transitional housing project in Denver, Colorado Established in 1974, Warren Village consists of two 100 unit apartment buildings located on two separate sites in a mixed-income neighborhood These facilities contain one-, two-, and three-bedroom unfurnished units (there are no congregate units), a daycare center, a job training program, commercial space, and administrative office space

After more than a decade of operation, Warren Village has a successful track record   Recent statistics show that the number of women employed rose from 47% upon entrance into the Village to 94% upon departure   Furthermore, the percentage of women receiving public assistance fell from 65% to 6%

Warren Village admits women who are 18 years of age and older and who have no more than four children under the age of 12   The women are re-ferred to Warren Village by local shelters, social service agencies, and churches   A diverse group of homeless women are served at Warren Village, including   battered women, deinstitutionalized women, and teenage mothers The diversity of the residents is one of the strengths of this program   For instance, women with parenting skills are often able to help teach childcare to

other residents   Each woman is interviewed upon admission to Warren Village, and then signs a contract detailing a plan of action   The maximum length of stay is two years, since it was found that beyond that time period women often have trouble leaving.

About 50% of the women living at the Village have children under the age of 12, making daycare an important component of this project   Each of the two facilities has a "Learning Center" to accommodate approximately 90-100 children   Warren Village manages these Learning Centers using city and state funds as well as volunteer help

As part of the Learning Center, Warren Village operates a computer training program using a donated Wang computer system   The women learn wordprocessing skills, job interviewing skills, resume writing, and filing   By providing training opportunities to the local business community, the Village is able to produce additional income for the program

The 10,000 square feet of commercial space is a commercial grade kitchen which is rented for use by local non-profit organizations   The commercial component has not been successful, in large part due to an oversupply of commercial space in the market area   The Executive Director of Warren Village indicated, however, that retail could be a very important addition to a transitional facility, particularly if it is linked to job training opportunities for residents   This arrangement generates income support and job training opportunities for residents   In developing this space, Warren Village was able to obtain federal funding by employing local residents

Warren Village has three full time staff and two live-in employees (one to handle building and maintenance, the other to assist residents)   Approximately 70 additional employees work under contract to provide counseling, job training, placement assistance, and childcare services

<u>Crossway Community</u>

Crossway Community is a transitional housing project currently under development in Wheaton, Maryland. The project involves the rehabilitation of a former school into 50 one- and two-bedroom unfurnished units The project will also include communal spaces for meeting rooms, laundry rooms, and administrative offices, as well as a daycare center to accommodate 40 children Currently the project is in the demolition phase, construction is scheduled to start in October 1986 and will take approximately one year to complete

Crossway Community is a program to assist to displaced homemakers, or those women with children who have suffered a radical loss of income due to divorce or widowhood It is expected that most of the women will not be AFDC recipients but rather will have some resources, however limited and insufficient Women will be referred through a local feeder network which is now being developed These women will be interviewed by an admissions committee and assisted in designing a personal program Maximum stay in the facility will be two years

In addition to daycare, this facility will offer a variety of family services including job development, parenting skills, and some health services The daycare center will be run by an agency which currently operates six other centers in Montgomery County Under this arrangement the County will pay the daycare teachers' salaries It is anticipated that only 6 staff members will be hired, including one live-in resident manager and one resident janitor

Funding for the project has come from a variety of sources including County funding for the rehabilitation work The school is leased from the County and the County acts as developer Federal and corporate funding is still being pursued The Community's board members, representatives from the business, government, and local communities, are expected to be helpful in obtaining additional resources

<u>Transitional Housing, Inc</u>

Transitional Housing, Inc (THI) in Cleveland, Ohio is located in a rehabilitated motel THI started operations in January 1986 and can accommodate one hundred single women in 45 efficiency apartments and 28 double occupancy units Currently, there are no facilities for children The women are referred to the project by a network of seven local temporary emergency shelters

Upon entering the program women are interviewed by the THI program coordinator A "residence agreement" is required of all women outlining either a job training or educational program which the woman agrees to participate Some classes are offered on-site but THI works with local agencies to avoid duplicating services The project has several meeting rooms for these classes

Current staff at THI includes a full-time program director, a part-time assistant, a full-time maintenance director, a finance director, and a resident tenant coordinator There is always one staff person on the grounds 24 hours a day, seven days a week

THI rehabilitation work was financed by a loan from a local bank This loan was backed up by private investors who loaned to THI at a point and a half below the bank's interest rate This difference in interest rates has provided several thousand dollars additional income The 45 efficiency units are paid for through Section 8 certificates, those living in the 28 congregate units pay roughly $100 per month

One of the strengths of this program is its location close to downtown and public transportation The facility also has a 70 car garage but it has not been able to generate income from this facility because of an insufficient demand for parking Perhaps the greatest drawback to this program is that it does not house children

THI is run by a Board consisting of two task forces - one to deal with housing issues, the other to handle the social services and educational issues Representative on the Board include community residents, local business-persons, and real estate brokers